Single Surgical Procedures 36

A Colour Atlas of

Mucosal Proctectomy and Ileal Reservoir Formation

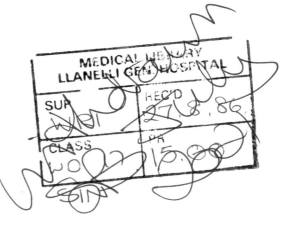

T. V. Taylor
MD, ChM, FRCS(Eng and Ed)
Consultant Surgeon, Manchester Royal Infirmary.

(Photography by University Department of Medical Illustration, Manchester Royal Infirmary.)

Wolfe Medical Publications Ltd
Year Book Medical Publishers, Inc

Published by Wolfe Medical Publications Ltd 1986
Printed by W.S. Cowell Ltd, 8 Buttermarket, Ipswich
United Kingdom
ISBN 0 7234 1053 4

This book is one of the titles in the series of
Wolfe Single Surgical Procedures, a series which
will eventually cover some 200 titles.

For a full list of Atlases in this series, plus
forthcoming titles and details of our surgical,
dental and veterinary Atlases, please write to
Wolfe Medical Publications Ltd, Wolfe House,
3 Conway Street, London W1P 6HE
or
Year Book Medical Publishers, Inc,
35 East Wacker Drive, Chicago, Ill. 60601

*Distributed in Continental North and Central
America, Hawaii and Puerto Rico by* Year Book
Medical Publishers, Inc

Library of Congress Cataloging-in-Publication Data

Taylor, T. Vincent.
A colour atlas of mucosal proctectomy and
ileal reservoir formation.

(Single surgical procedures series; vol. 36).
Includes index.
1. Rectum—Surgery—Atlases.
2. Ulcerative colitis—Surgery—Atlases.
3. Mucous membrane—Surgery—Atlases.
4. Ileum—Surgery—Atlases.   I. Title.
II. Series: Single surgical procedures series: v. 36.
[DNLM: 1. Colitis, Ulcerative—surgery—atlases.
2. Rectum—surgery—atlases. WI 17 T246cd]
RD544.T39 1986   617′.5547   86–4127
ISBN 0–8151–8747–5

We list below a few of the other titles in print and in
preparation in the Single Surgical Procedures series. For a
comprehensive list please write.

Published
Parotidectomy
Traditional Meniscectomy
Inguinal Hernias & Hydroceles in Infants and Children
Surgery for Pancreatic & Associated Carcinomata
Subtotal Thyroidectomy
Anterior Resection of Rectum
Boari Bladder-Flap Procedure
Surgery for Varicose Veins
Treatment of Carpal Tunnel Syndrome
Seromyotomy for Chronic Duodenal Ulcer
Surgery for Undescended Testes
Operations on the Internal Carotid Artery
Renal Transplant
Lumbar Discography
Visceral Artery Reconstruction
Flexor Tendon Repair
Proctocolectomy
Common Operations of the Foot
Right Hemicolectomy
Extra-cranial and Intra-cranial Anastomosis
Surgery for Hirschsprung's Disease
Thyroid Lobectomy
Surgery at the Thoracic Outlet
External Fixation
Anterior Cervical Spine Fusion
Liver Transplantation
Modified Radical Mastectomy
Paratopic Transplant of Body and Tail of the Pancreas
Subdiaphragmatic Total Gastrectomy for Malignant Disease
Rupture of the Rotator Cuff
Left Hemicolectomy

In Production
Surgery of Lymphoedema of the Lower Limbs
Gastric Revision Operations
Plastering Techinques
Cleft Lip Surgery
Mastectomy with Immediate Reconstruction
Joint Replacement of the Hand
Periodontal Surgery

Some Future Titles
Biliary Enteric Anastomosis with Strictures in Common Bile Duct
Surgical Disencumberment of the Thoracic Outlet
Aortic Endarterectomy
Axillary Dissection for Melanoma
Groin Dissection for Melanoma
Coronary Artery Bypass
Omental Transposition
Orthopaedic Hip Approaches
Management of Venous Disease
Upper Thoracic Sympathectomy
Inguinal Hernia Repair
Vascular Access
Dental Analgesia
Hiatus Hernia
Plastic and Reconstructive Surgery
Occlusion/Malocclusion
Femoral and Tibial Osteotomy
Resection of Aortic Aneurysm
Ileo-Rectal Anastomosis
Techniques of Nerve Grafting and Repair
Surgery for Dupuytren's Contracture
Athrodesis of the Ankle
Spondylolisthesis
Repair of Prolapsed Rectum
Splenectomy
Anterior Nephrectomy
Caecocystoplasty
Total Gastrectomy
Billroth 1 Gastrectomy
Billroth 2 Gastrectomy
Abdominal Incisions
Thoracotomy
Appendicectomy
Incisional Hernia
Lung Lobectomy
Lung Removal
Haemorrhoids
Rectosigmoid Resection
Surgery for Anorectal Incontinence
Visceral Vascular Occlusion
Aortofemoral Bypass
Aortoilac Disobliteration
Joint Replacement of Wrist and Hand
Operative Fixation of Fractures of the Forearm
Minor Operative Procedures
Technique of Arthroscopy of the Knee

Contents

Introduction

The surgical treatment of ulcerative colitis began at the turn of the century when Weir (1902) of New York performed an appendicostomy, an operation first suggested by Keetly of London in 1895. The operation continued to be performed until 1940. Ileostomy provided complete faecal diversion from the colon and after 1940 became more popular than appendicostomy. It was soon realised, however, that faecal diversion was not adequate to produce remission of the disease. By the 1950s surgeons were recommending the addition of colectomy. Subtotal colectomy was later replaced, in most centres, by the performance of procto-colectomy. The latter was the first totally curative operation which obviated any subsequent risk of malignancy and was often associated with improvement, if not complete cure, of the non-gastro-intestinal manifestations of the disorder. In addition to the problems associated with a permanent ileostomy, proctocolectomy may be complicated by impotence, bladder dysfunction and chronic persistent perineal sinus. It is, however, the desire to achieve intestinal continence which has led surgeons to strive for improved procedures, firstly ileorectal anastomosis, later the Kock continent ileostomy and more recently mucosal proctectomy, ileal reservoir formation and ileo-anal anastomosis.

The potential advantage of the latter over other operations for ulcerative colitis is that, while curing the disorder, the operation restores gastro-intestinal continuity and continence and eliminates the need for an ileostomy. Additionally the pelvic autonomic nerves are less likely to be damaged, and bladder and sexual dysfunction may be prevented.

The concept underlying the operation was initiated by Ravitch and Sabiston in 1947 who performed experiments in the dog. In the following year Ravitch performed the operation on two young adults with ulcerative colitis but did not create an ileal reservoir. Other surgeons performing the technique at this time described problems, chiefly of sepsis and incontinence. It has been known for over 20 years, following the work of Soave in children with Hirschprung's disease, that continence could consistently be achieved after removal of the rectal mucosa. Several workers achieved continence after ileo-anal anastomosis with mucosal proctectomy, but frequency of bowel action was a problem. This has, to some extent, been overcome by the use of an ileal reservoir, first used experimentally in dogs in 1955. Parks and Nicholls in 1978 combined a triple loop ileal pouch with a mucosal proctectomy for ulcerative colitis and an ever-increasing number of surgeons have investigated the technique since then, most notably Kelly at the Mayo Clinic and Johnston in Leeds. In recent years the major modification to the triplicated Parks pouch has been the J-pouch introduced by Utsonomiya (1980). This pouch is illustrated here.

Indications for surgery in ulcerative colitis

Failure of medical treatment to control the disorder resulting in intractability and chronic invalidism is the major indication for surgical intervention. The risk of malignant change is greatest in those with total colitis of over 20 years duration. Annual colonoscopic assessment of the disease should be carried out in those whose disease has been active for over ten years, particularly when total colonic involvement is present. The presence of epithelial dysplasia on colonoscopic biopsy is often a heralding sign of the subsequent development of malignancy which may be used as an indication for surgery. Severe non-gastrointestinal manifestations of the disorder such as pyoderma gangrenosa, severe joint manifestations or eye complications frequently respond well to surgical treatment of the colitis. The development of toxic dilatation of the colon is an indication for emergency surgery.

Indications for mucosal proctectomy

All patients requiring surgery for ulcerative colitis may be considered for mucosal proctectomy, with the proviso that an upper age limit might become obligatory. Only with increasing experience of the technique will this become apparent, and even then some flexibility will be required, but this limit may be as low as 50 years.

Absolute contra-indications to performance of the operation are:

1 A pre-operative diagnosis of Crohn's disease;
2 The presence of rectal carcinoma;

3 Pre-operative anal incontinence;
4 Coexisting medical conditions making major surgery hazardous.

Acute toxic dilatation of the colon is not a contra-indication to the ultimate performance of a mucosal proctectomy, which can be carried out at a later date following an emergency total colectomy.

It is the author's practice to describe both the principles of mucosal proctectomy and panproctocolectomy with ileostomy to the patient who is referred for surgical treatment of their ulcerative colitis. The more time-consuming and more difficult nature of the former is emphasised at the same time as the definite aesthetic advantages over the latter. In my experience, most of these patients, often young women, elect to undergo mucosal proctectomy.

It is possible that mucosal proctectomy may supersede ileorectal anastomosis in patients with familial polyposis coli but further experience of the operation is required before most surgeons would adopt the procedure.

Pre-operative preparation

The patient should be well hydrated and any abnormality in the concentration of serum electrolytes should be corrected. If the patient's haemoglobin concentration is less than 10 g/dl pre-operative blood transfusion should be given, if possible more than 24 hours prior to surgery. Where malnutrition is present a period of enteral or even parenteral hyperalimentation may be necessary. If nutrition remains inadequate then colectomy and ileostomy should be carried out reserving the performance of mucosal proctectomy to a later date when the nutritional state has been corrected. An intensive course of topical rectal steroid enemata is valuable in improving the inflammation in the rectal mucosa prior to mucosal proctectomy.

Because of the severe diarrhoea which is usually present in the patient undergoing surgery for ulcerative colitis, aggressive mechanical preparation of the bowel is particularly distressing and unnecessary. It is useful, however, to use half the recommended dose of sodium picosulphate followed by one phosphate enema which achieves good mechanical clearance in these patients.

Per-operative broad spectrum intravenous antibiotics should be given in divided doses over a 24-hour period. An aminoglycoside along with metronidazole (500 mg 8 hourly) is a suitable combination. The first dose should be given at the time of induction of anaesthesia. As the patient will, in all probability, have been receiving systemic steroids up to the time of surgery, during the operative period and first few postoperative days hydrocortisone 100 mg intravenously 6 hourly should be given. Six units of blood should be cross matched. Once the patient is anaesthetised a urethral catheter is inserted and the rectum is washed out with aqueous povidone iodine.

Postoperative management

Following the operation, which will next be described in detail, the patient is transferred to the recovery area where a series of careful observations are made of the pulse, blood pressure, respiratory rate, temperature and urine output. The loop ileostomy normally functions between the second and fourth postoperative day at which time the nasogastric tube is removed and oral fluids are commenced.

I usually remove the urinary and pouch catheters on about the fifth or sixth postoperative day, by which time the patient is taking a light diet. All being well, discharge from hospital is arranged for about the twelfth postoperative day. On out-patient review at one month, particular attention is paid to the stoma; I perform a digital examination of the pouch, gently dilating any degree of stenosis. At four months the pouch is examined radiologically and endoscopically prior to closing the loop ileostomy.

Operative technique

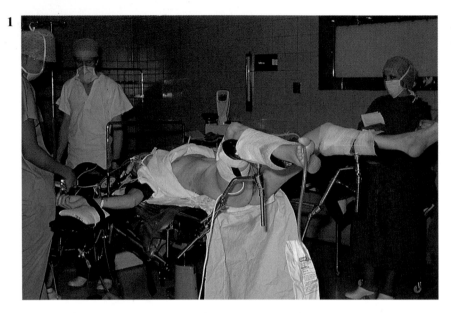

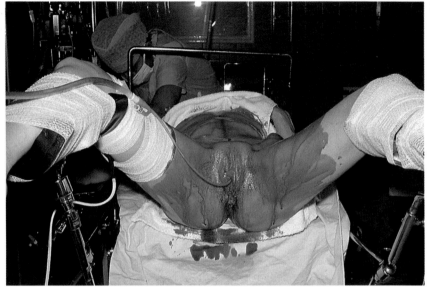

1 **The patient is positioned supine on the operating table with the hips in flexion and abduction using the Lloyd Davies supports.** A pillow is placed under the sacrum and the table is adjusted to a Trendelenburg tilt of 10–15°.

2 **The whole abdomen, perineum and proximal thighs are sterilised with povidone iodine solution.**

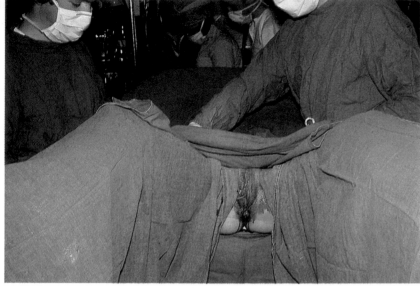 3

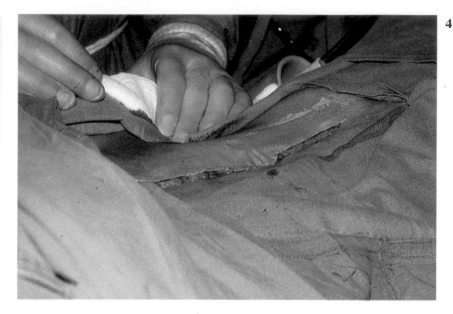 4

3 **Drapes are applied to expose the whole of the midline of the abdomen and perineum.**

4 **The abdomen is opened through a long midline incision skirting the umbilicus.** An alternative approach is through a long left paramedian rectus-displacing incision, extending from the pubis almost to the costal margin.

5 **The incision is deepened and haemostasis is secured.**

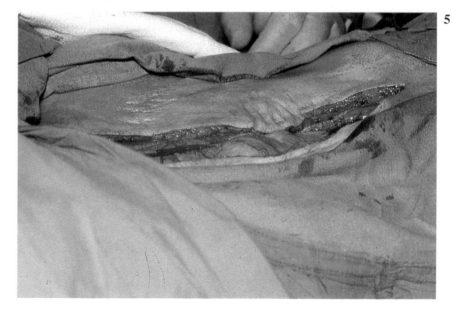 5

6

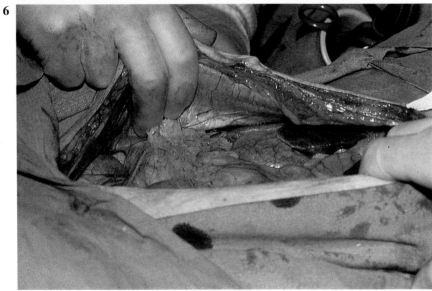

7

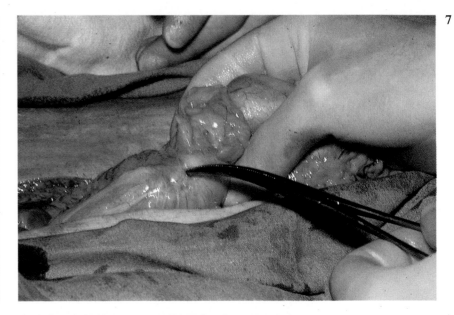

6 A laparotomy is performed, inspecting all of the abdominal viscera.

7 The colon is inspected in detail to ensure that there is no evidence of malignancy within it. The characteristic appearance of the serosal surface of the bowel is of inflammation or serositis, with increased vascularity due to leashes of fine tortuous vessels coursing across it. Multiple small ecchymoses are often present.

8 Detailed inspection of the liver is carried out to exclude inflammatory or neoplastic disease associated with ulcerative colitis.

8

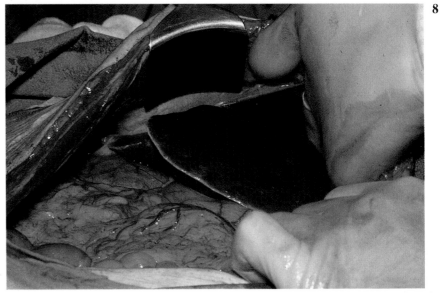

9

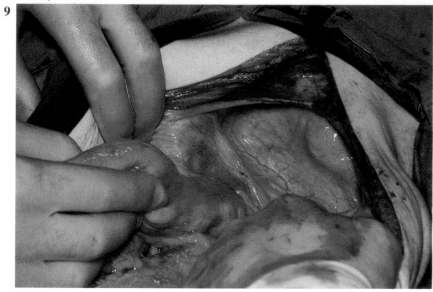

10

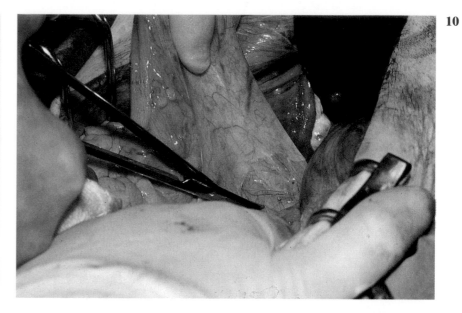

11

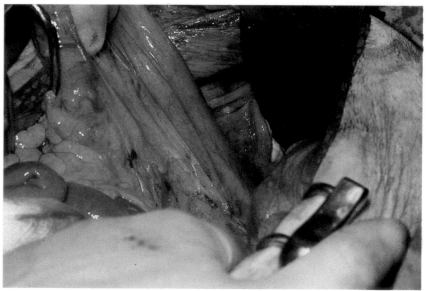

9   The pelvis is exposed before starting the dissection.

10   **Gentle upward and left lateral traction is applied to the sigmoid and rectal mesocolon.** An incision is made on the right side of the base of the rectal mesentery.

11   **The incision in the peritoneum is continued down to the level of the peritoneal reflection.**

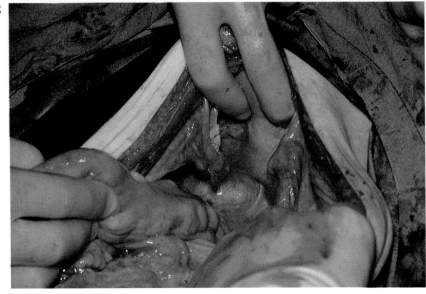

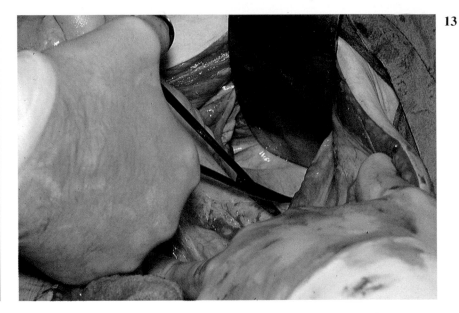

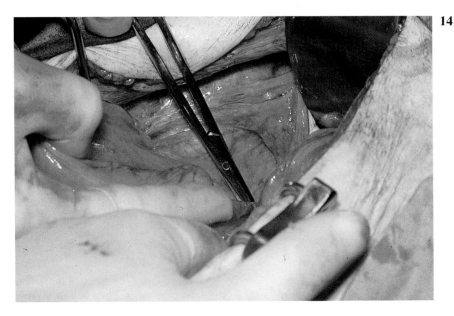

12   The pouch of Douglas is now exposed.

13   **The peritoneal incision is continued around the front of the rectum in the pouch of Douglas.** This incision is facilitated by placing the peritoneal fold under gentle traction.

14   **The peritoneum is here being incised at the level of its reflection.**

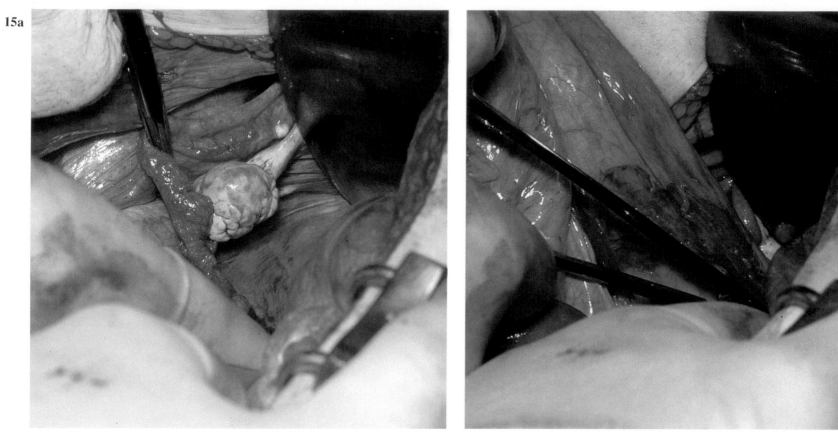

15a and 15b Further mobilisation of the upper rectum is achieved by blunt dissection and by using dissecting scissors.

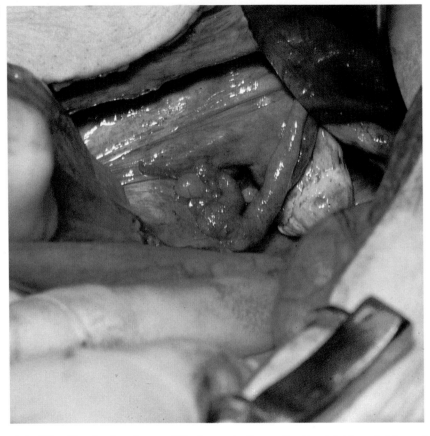

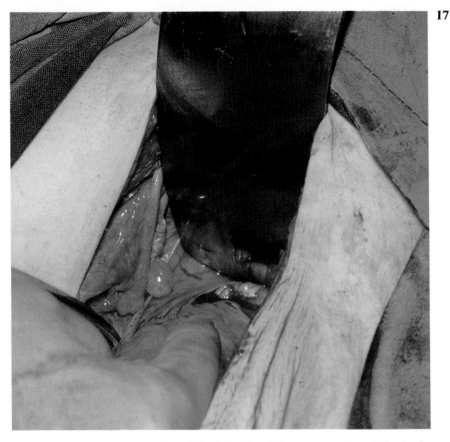

16 The distal colon is now lifted over to the patient's right hand side and gentle upward traction is applied.

17 The peritoneal reflection of the left side of the upper rectum is incised.

Caution: The left ureter should be carefully avoided. It lies medial and superficial to the common iliac artery at its bifurcation. That a given structure is the ureter can be ascertained by gently swabbing it and producing the characteristic peristaltic movement.

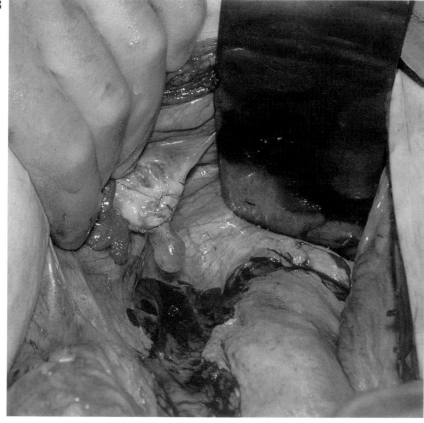

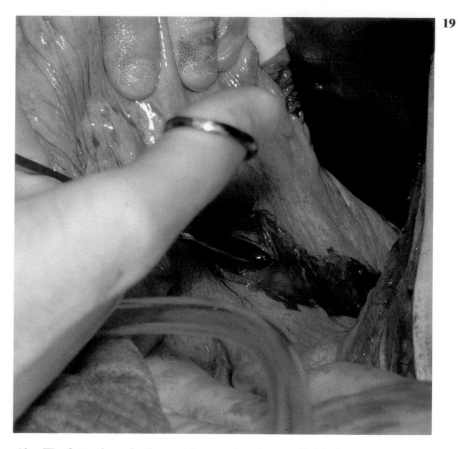

18　The peritoneum has now been incised around the whole of the upper rectum and its mesentery.

19　The fatty tissue in the rectal mesentery is now divided.

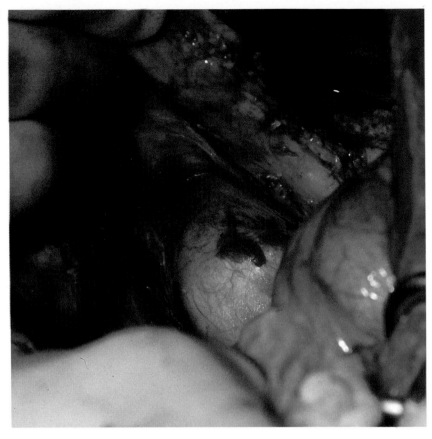

20 Blunt dissection is used to expose the presacral space.

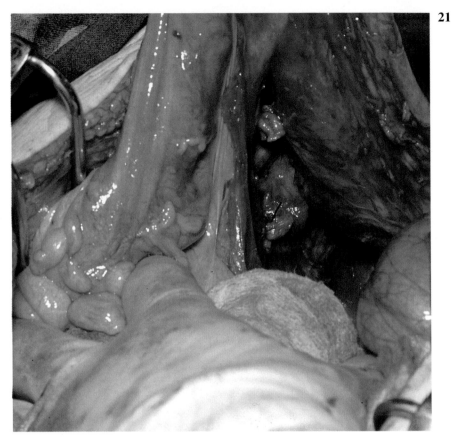

21 This dissection is continued to mobilise the posterior rectum down to the sacrococcygeal area.

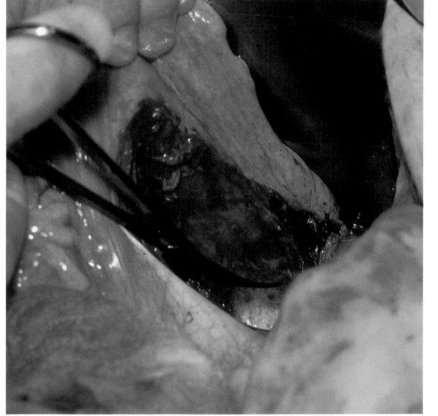
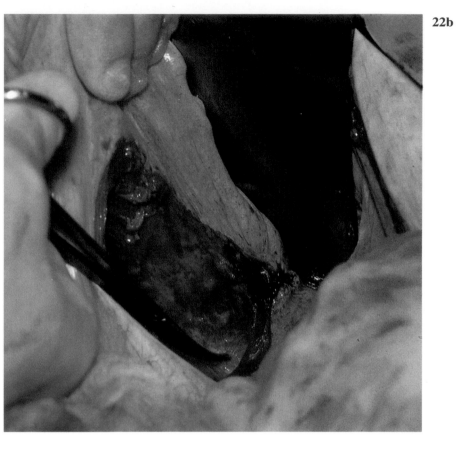

22a and 22b Further mobilisation of the posterior rectal wall from the presacral area.

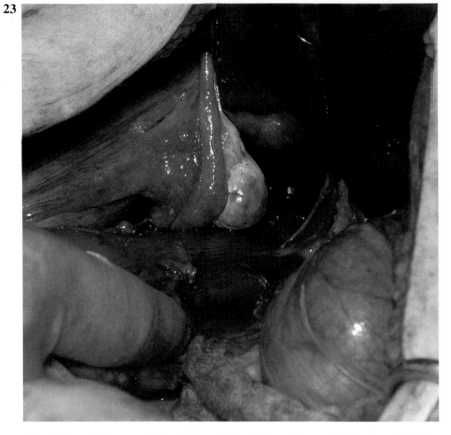

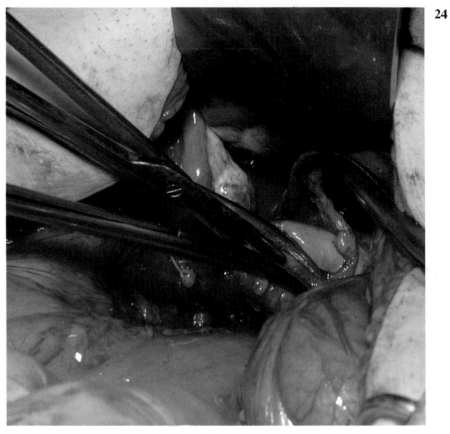

23   The anterior rectal wall is mobilised from the posterior aspect of the vagina. A deep pelvic retractor is useful here to lift the bladder forwards. This mobilisation is best achieved by cautious dissection with scissors.

24   Small vessels in the rectal mesentery are divided.

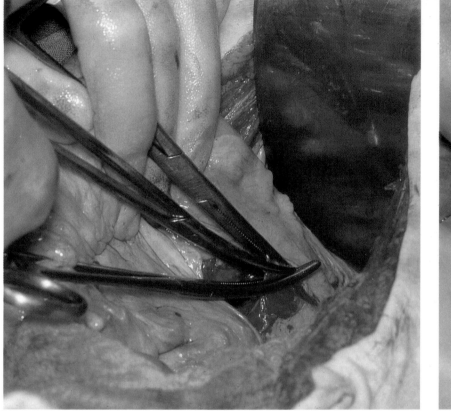
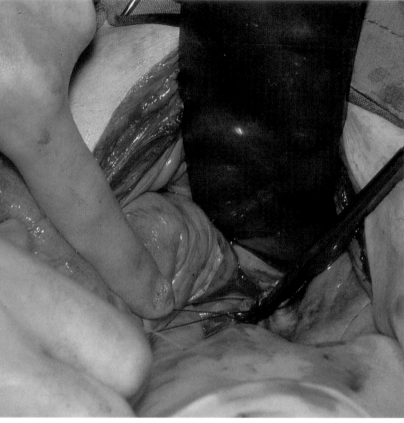

25a and **25b** **The rectum has now been freed posteriorly and anteriorly.**
It remains attached on either side by the lateral ligaments. The right
lateral ligament is now divided and ligated (**25b**).

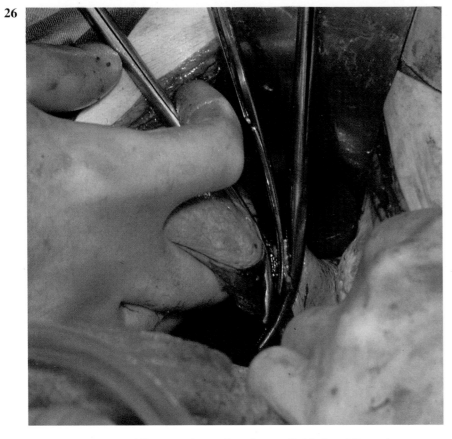

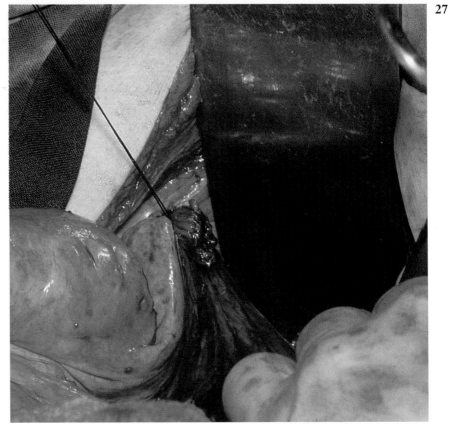

26 The left lateral ligament is rendered taut, divided and ligated.

27 Following division of the lateral ligaments the rectum is retracted proximally.

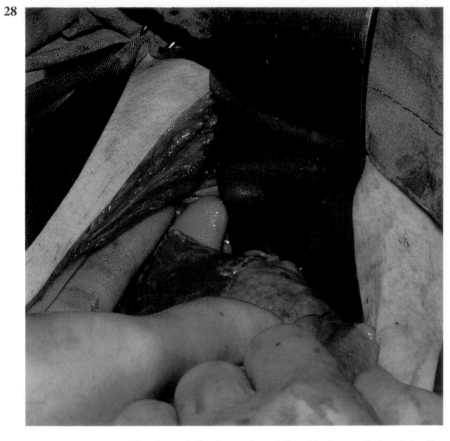

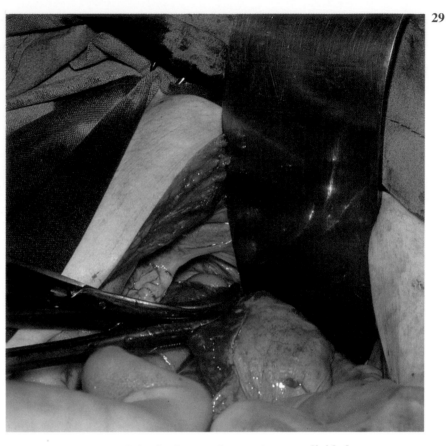

28 Further mobilisation of the lateral rectal walls is carried out to the level of the musculature of the pelvic floor.

29 Any vessels remaining in the rectal mesentery are divided.

30 The surgeon's view of the pelvic floor.

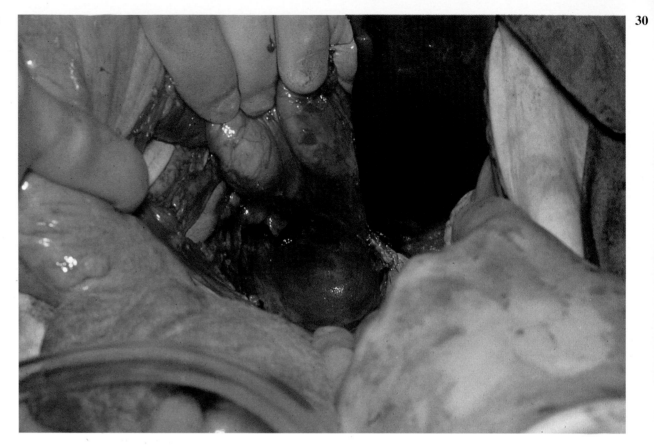

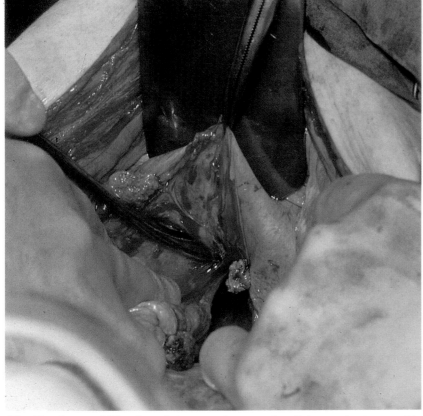

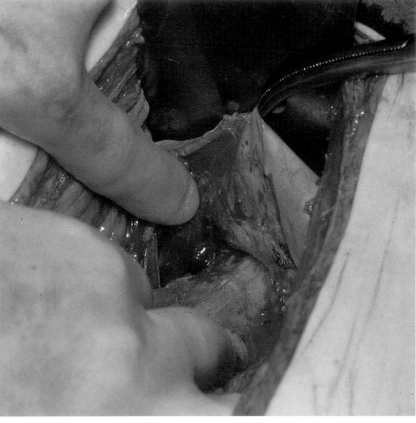

31 Further mobilisation of the anterior rectal wall is required to enable the rectum to be everted into the perineum.

32 Completed exposure of the anterior rectal wall.

33 The pelvic floor on completion of the rectal dissection. The rectum in the upper part of the figure is pulled taut.

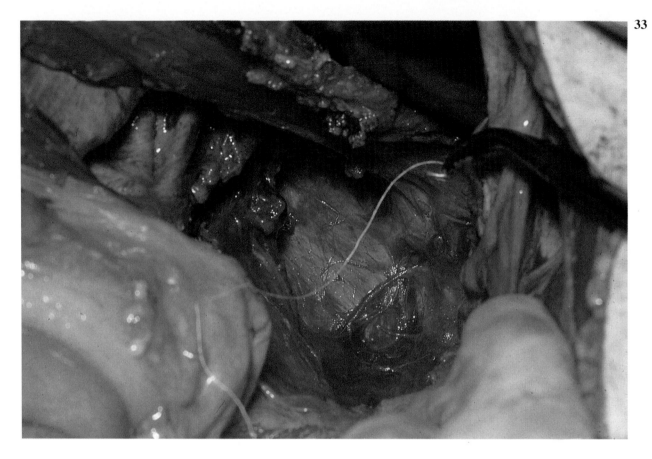

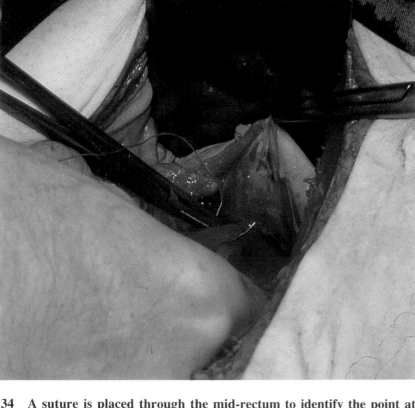

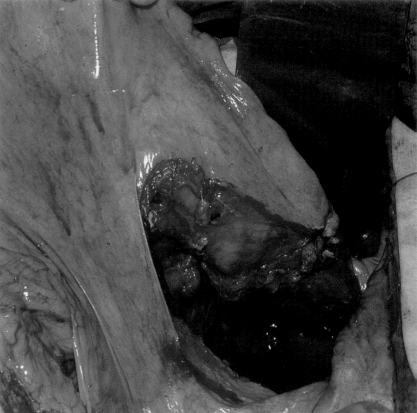

34 A suture is placed through the mid-rectum to identify the point at which the rectum is to be divided. This is approximately 7 cm from the anal verge. The point is measured by requesting that an assistant insert a finger in the rectum.

35 The lower sigmoid colon is lifted out of the wound prior to division of its mesentery.

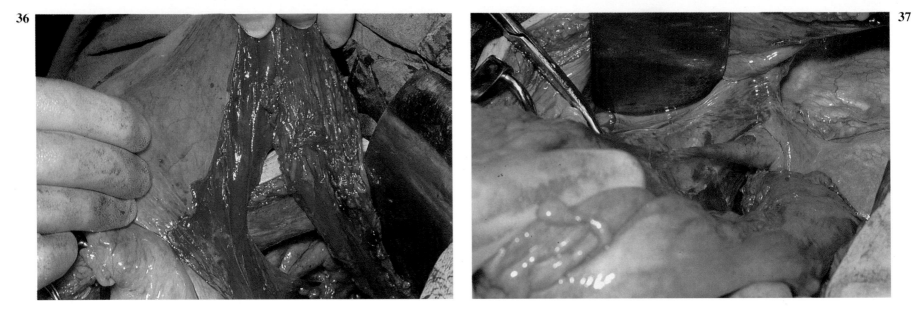

36 Mobilisation of the sigmoid colon is carried out.

37 Pulling the sigmoid colon over to the patient's right, the peritoneal reflection in the left paracolic gutter is divided to free the sigmoid in a medial direction.

38 The inferior mesenteric vessels now require division.

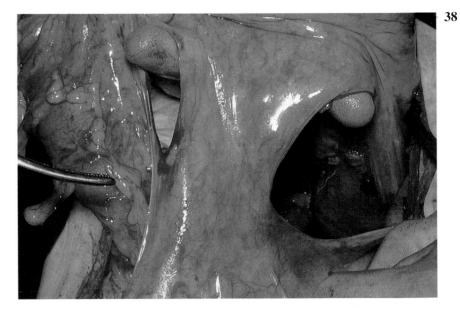

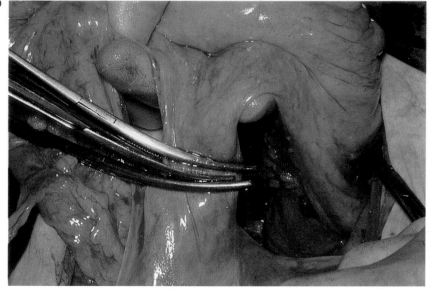

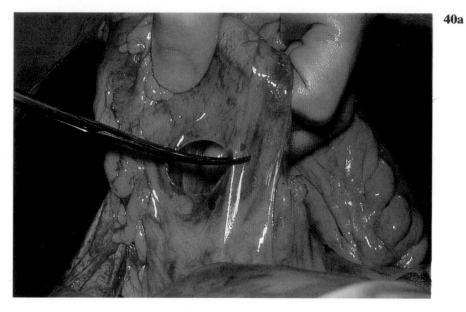

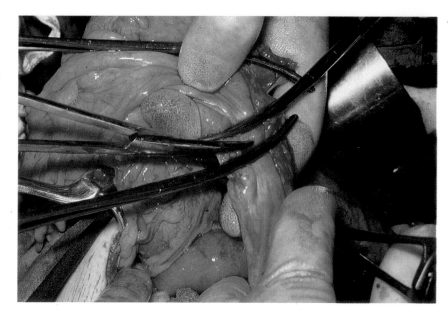

39 These vessels are clamped and divided close to their origin.

Caution: Identify the left ureter to ensure that it is not damaged.

40a and 40b The mesentery of the sigmoid colon is further mobilised in a proximal direction.

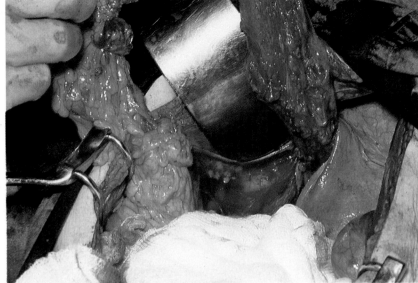

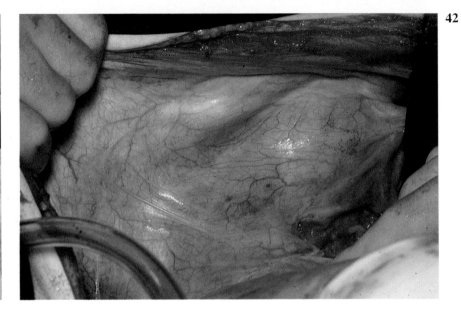

41 The sigmoid colon along with the upper and middle rectum now lie free.

42 The upper left paracolic gutter is exposed.

43 The base of the colonic mesentery along the left paracolic gutter is incised.

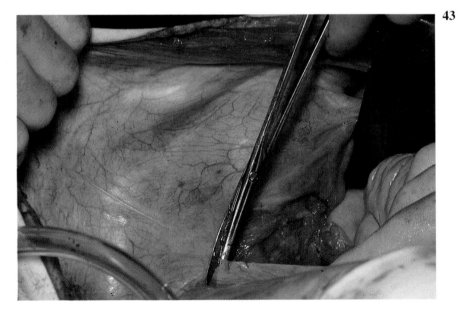

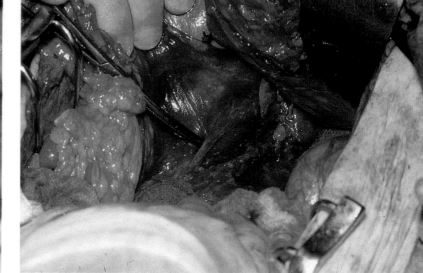

44 The splenic flexure of the colon is retracted caudally and the spleno-colic ligament is incised.

45 The mesentery of the descending colon is reflected towards the midline. The left ureter is again identified so that it is not endangered in this part of the dissection.

46 The vessels in the mesentery of the descending colon are now clamped, divided and ligated.

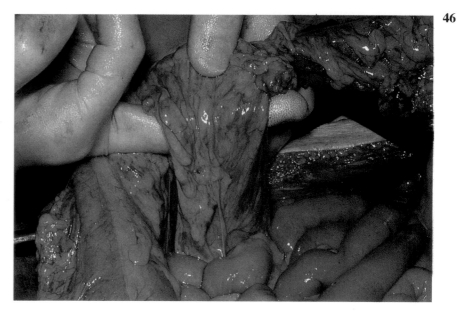

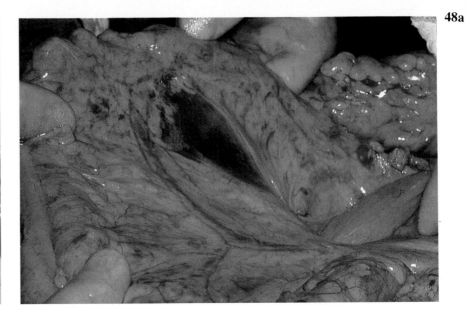

47   The splenic flexure and the left side of the transverse colon can now be delivered into the wound.

48a to 48e   The middle colic vessels are divided and ligated.

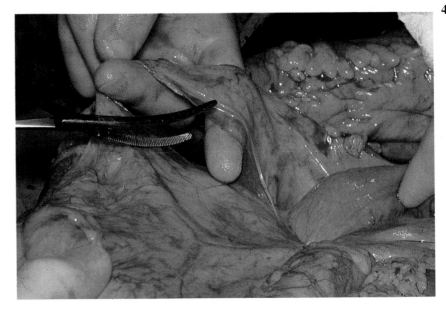

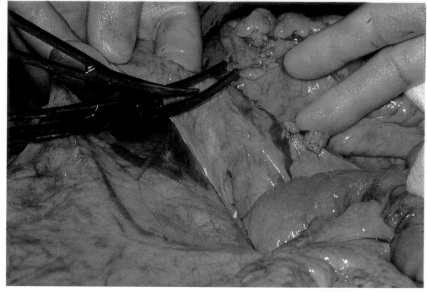

48c

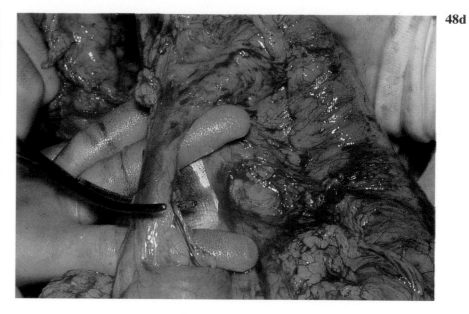

48d

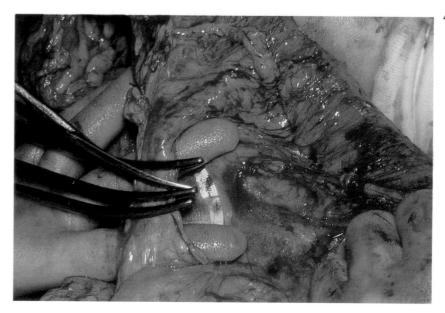

48e

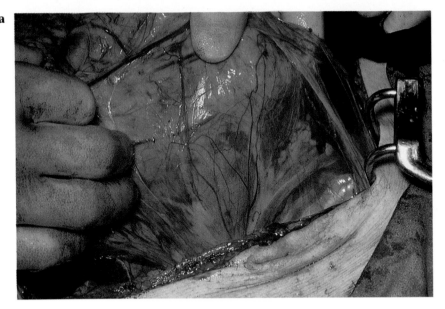

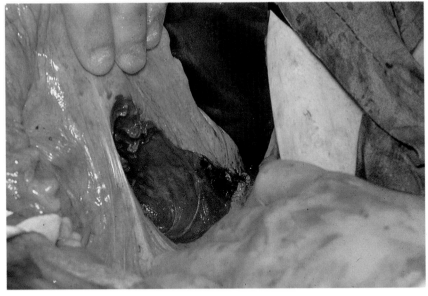

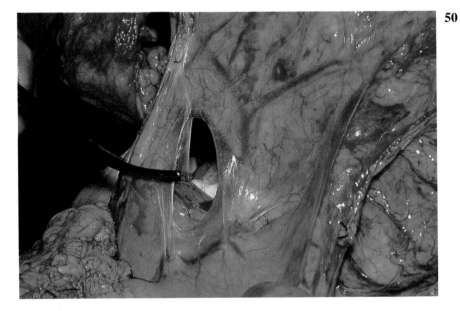

49a and 49b The colonic mesentery along the right paracolic gutter is incised from below the caecum to just above the hepatic flexure.

50 The hepatocolic ligament is divided in order to free the hepatic flexure of the colon.

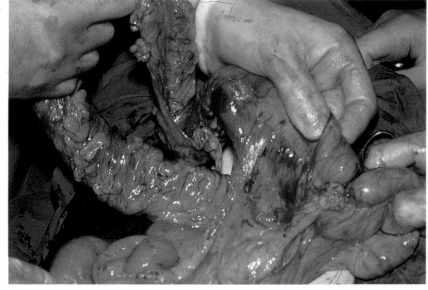

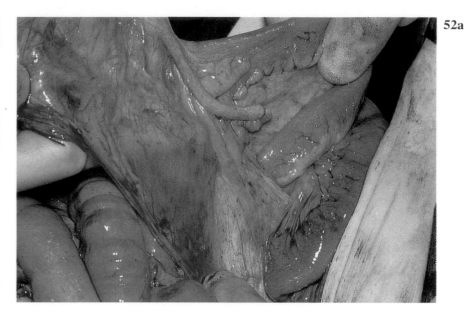

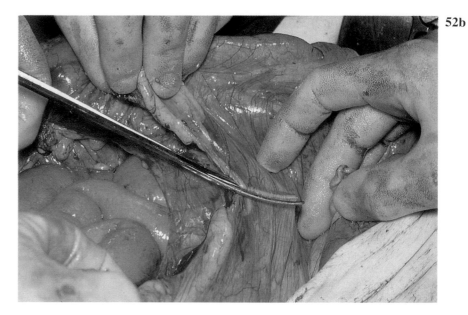

51 The right side of the colon can now be lifted out of the abdomen.

Caution: Be careful not to damage either the right ureter, the duodenum or the spermatic or ovarian vessels.

52a and 52b The appendix and terminal ileum are lifted out of the peritoneal cavity prior to division of the ileocolic and right colic vessels.

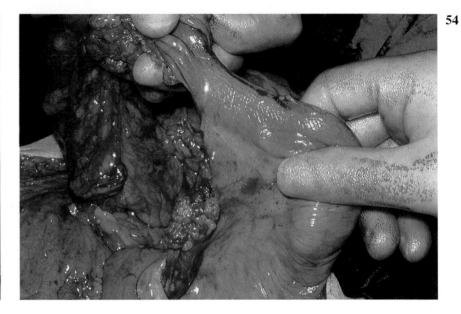

53 The terminal ileal mesenteric vascular arcades are divided.

54 The ileum is preserved to within approximately 1–2 cm of the ileocaecal junction.

55 Occlusion clamps are applied to the terminal ileum.

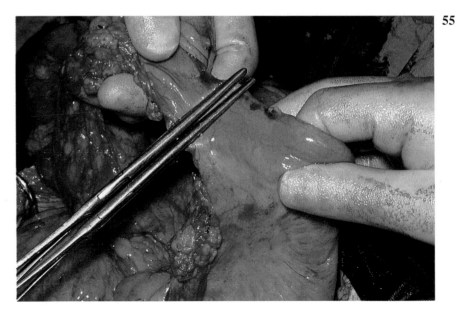

56 The ileum is now prepared for division.

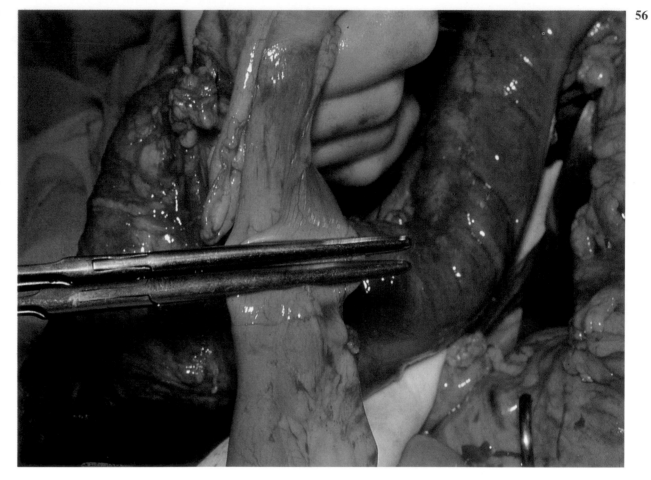

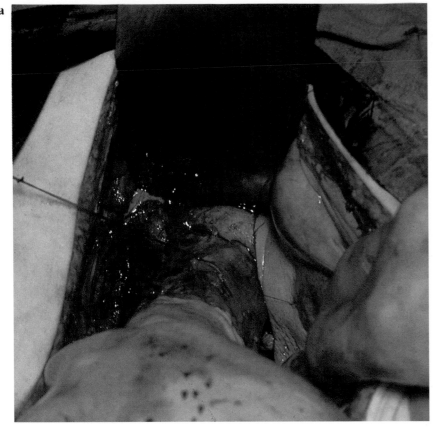

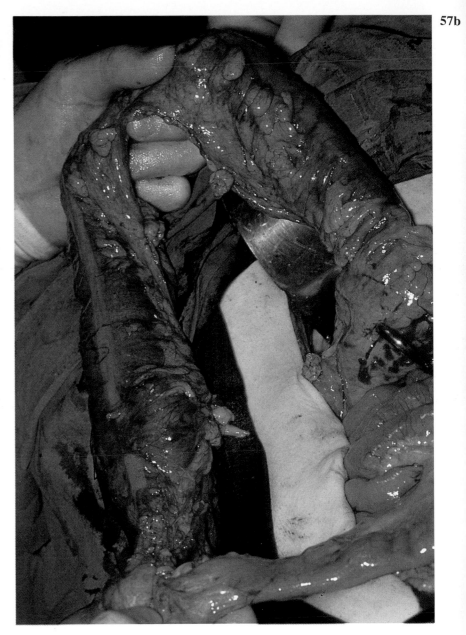

57a and 57b   The whole colon from the middle rectum (a) to the terminal ileum (b) has now been mobilised.

58 A right angled light occlusion clamp is applied to the middle rectum, approximately 7 cm from the anal verge, where the rectum is to be divided. This level is assessed by asking the assistant to insert a finger into the rectum and measure the level of division.

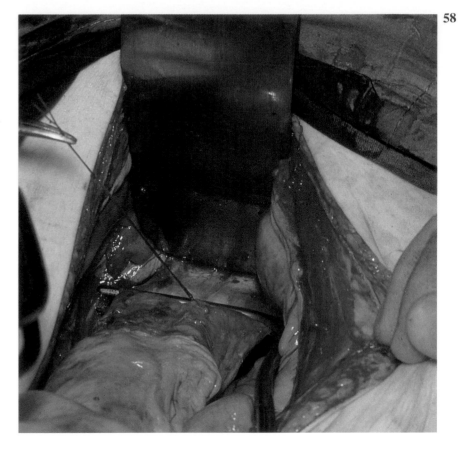

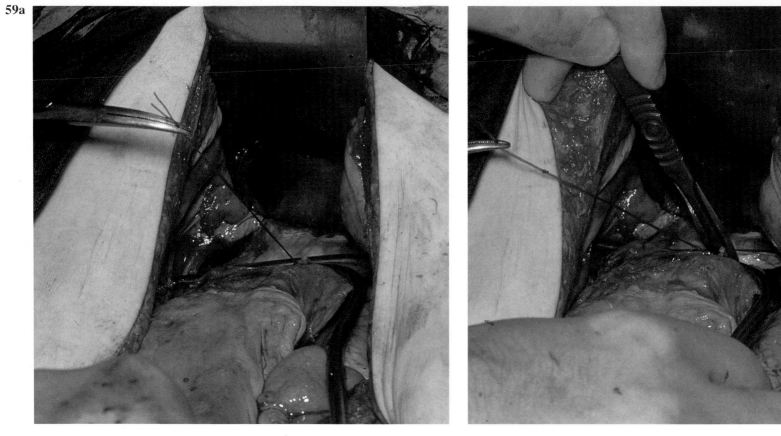

59a and 59b A second right-angled clamp is applied directly above the first and the rectum is divided between the two clamps.

60 The terminal ileum is divided and the whole colon together with the upper and middle rectum are removed.

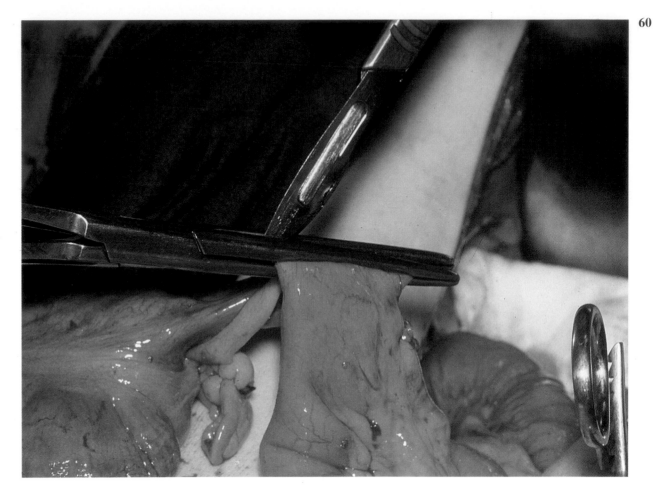

61

62

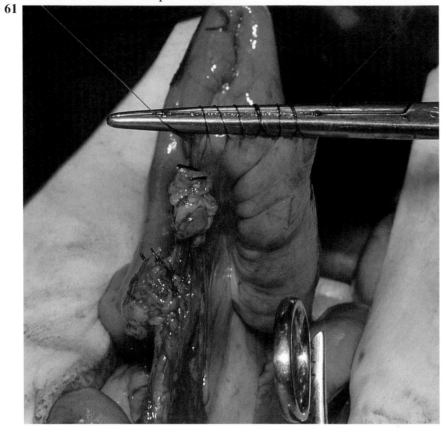

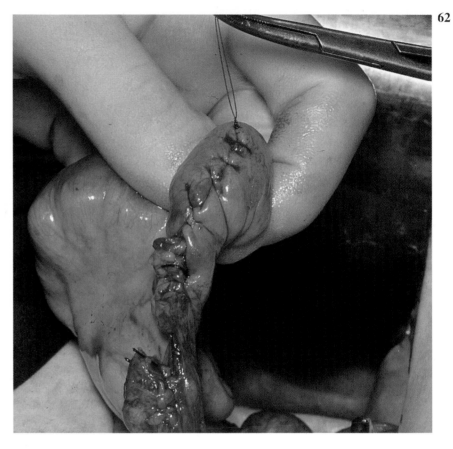

61 The terminal ileum is oversewn with an absorbable suture (PDS).

62 A two-layer closure is performed, burying the first layer of full-thickness sutures by a seromuscular layer.

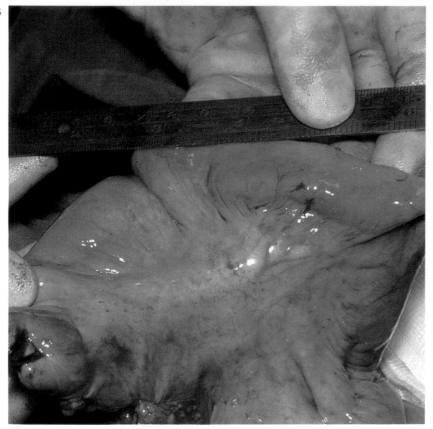

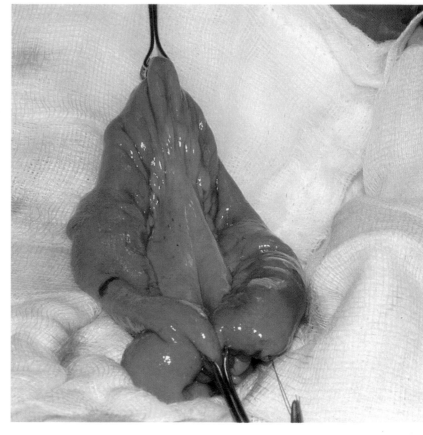

63 A 15 cm length of terminal ileum is measured.

64 Two equal 15 cm limbs are apposed for creation of the ileal pouch.
The technique of creating a 'J' shaped pouch will be shown, the
alternative being to manufacture a Park's pouch using three parallel
lengths of ileum.

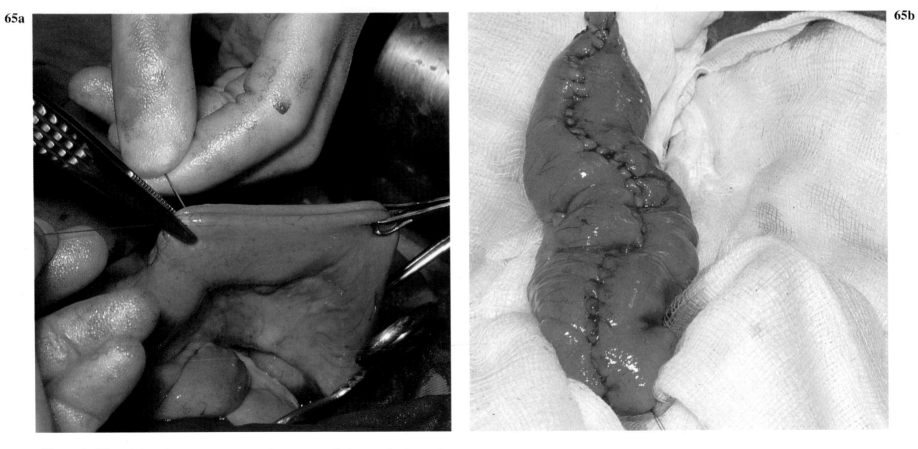

65a and 65b A continuous seromuscular suture is inserted along the 15 cm length of the antimesenteric border of the two limbs of ileum.

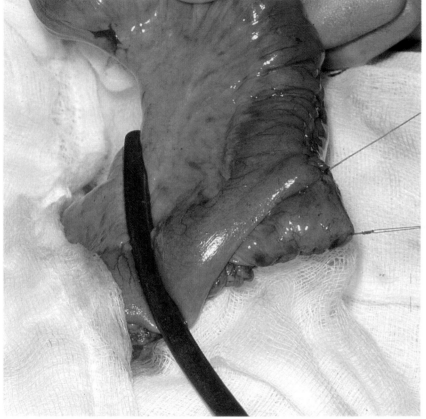

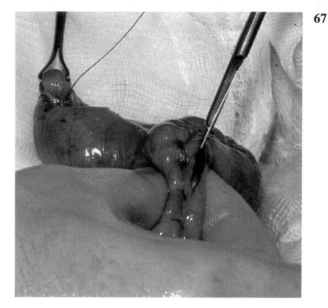

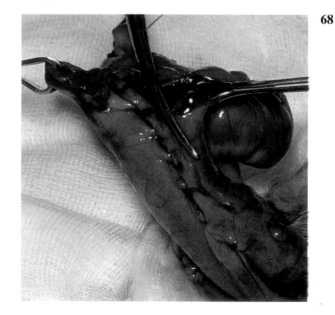

66 A light occlusion clamp is placed across the ileal mesentery to prevent excessive bleeding after division of the bowel wall.

67 An incision is made into the ileal lumen on either side of the seromuscular suture.

68 Both loops of ileum are incised along the whole length of the pouch.

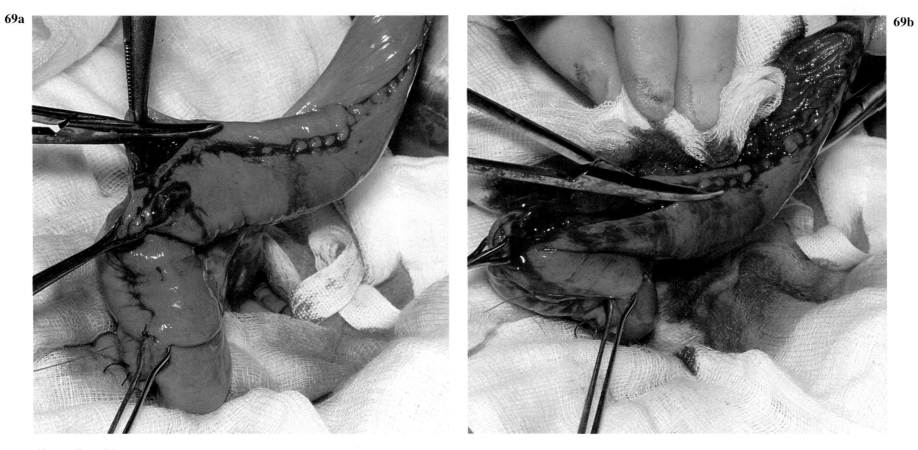

69a to 69c   The two lengths of ileum are laid open.

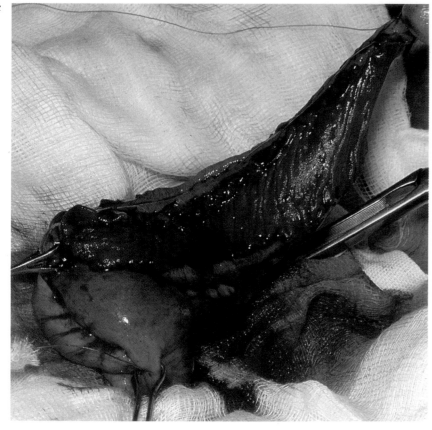

69c

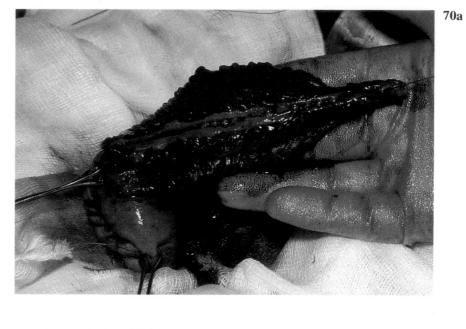

70a

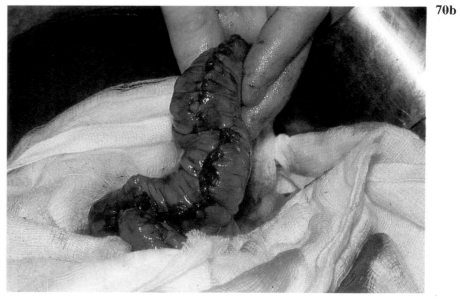

70b

70a and 70b   A full thickness continuous absorbable suture is placed
along the whole length of the pouch.

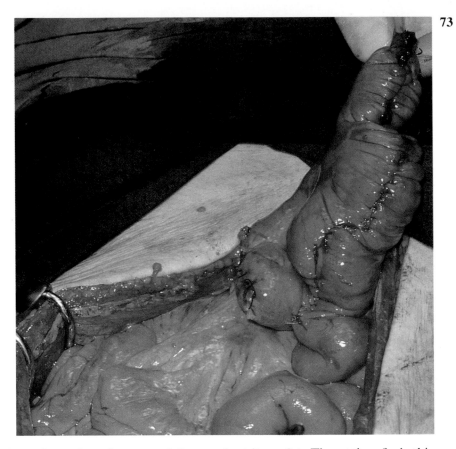

71 A de Pezzer catheter is put into the apex of the pouch at its outlet. The author finds this helpful, as it facilitates the positioning of the pouch in the denuded rectum, the approximation of the mucosal surfaces and ultimately the performance of the anastomosis.

72 The seromuscular layer is completed.

73 The pouch can be seen to be suspended from a long mesentery, allowing its apex to reach well down into the pelvis. Achieving an adequate length so that the apex of the pouch can reach the anorectal junction is crucial to the success of the procedure. This can pose problems particularly in the short and relatively obese patient. Where difficulty is encountered increased length of the pouch may be provided by: (i) mobilising the superior mesenteric artery back to its origin, (ii) creating 'windows' in the mesentery between the arcades of the mesenteric vessels, (iii) dividing the terminal branches to the apex of the pouch.

Performance of the mucosal proctectomy

There are two approaches available for the performance of the mucosal proctectomy. In the first illustrated, in which the Park's anal retractor is used, the mucosa is removed with the lower rectum in situ. In the second technique the rectum, which has been completely mobilised, is prolapsed through the anal verge allowing the mucosa to be removed from outside of the anus. This technique permits easier resection of the mucosa but requires lower dissection and more extensive mobilisation of the rectum **with a potentially greater risk of impotence in the male, and bladder dysfunction.**

Dissection of the mucosa with the rectum in situ

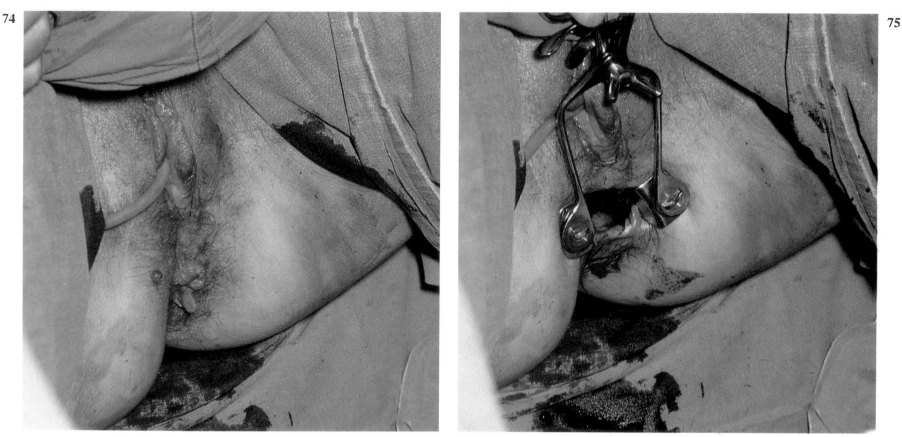

74   **The perineum is prepared for the mucosal proctectomy.**

75   **The anus is manually dilated using four fingers.** The Park's retractor is inserted.

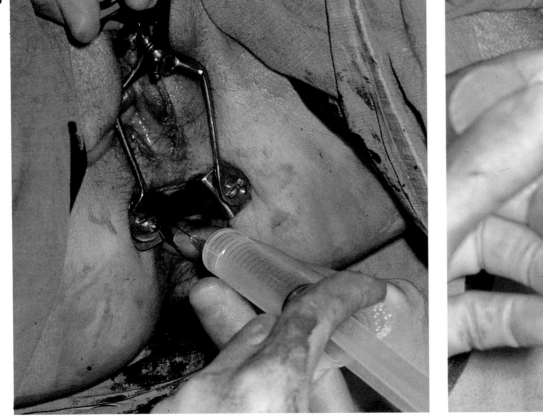

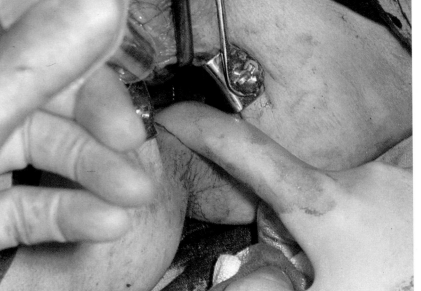

76 A 1:300,000 solution of adrenaline is injected beneath the rectal mucosa. This elevates the mucosa from the submucosa, making the dissection easier to perform.

77 A Langenbeck retractor is placed in the lower rectum. This facilitates the exposure required to dissect the mucosa off the submucosal tissues.

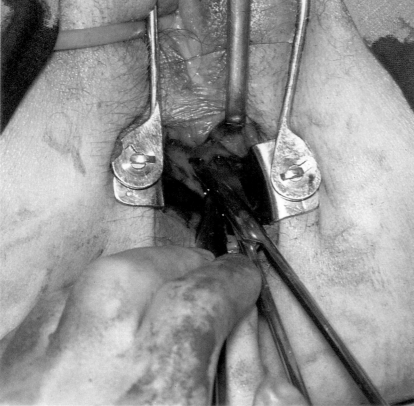

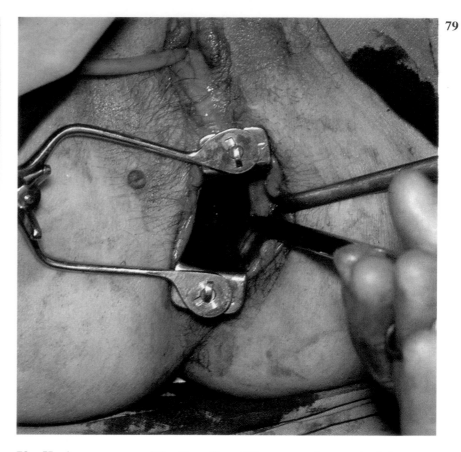

78 Using dissecting forceps to lift the mucosa off the rectal wall the dissecting scissors are inserted beneath the mucosa and into the submucosal plane.

79 Having commenced the dissection of the mucosa in a vertical plane the Park's retractor is rotated to allow exposure of the lateral rectal walls.

80 The mucosa is gradually elevated off the submucosa, using dissecting scissors to separate it carefully.

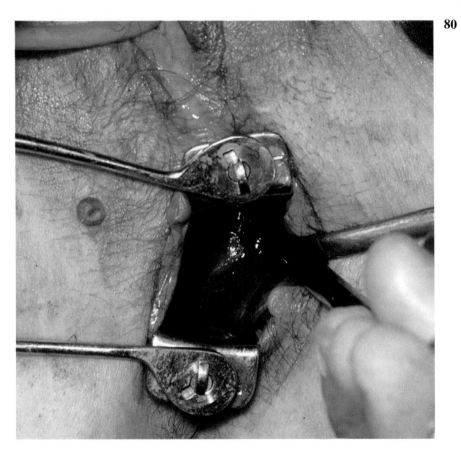

81

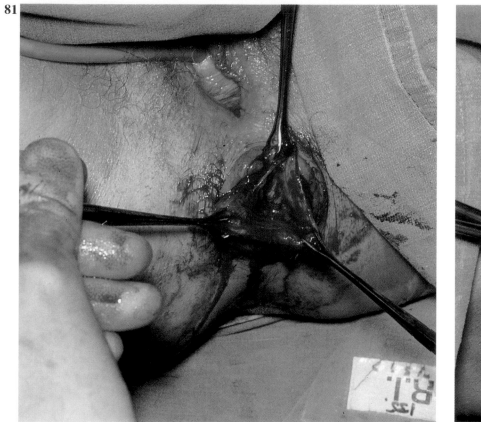

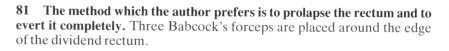

82

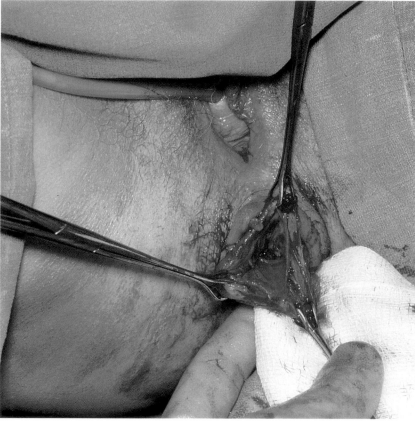

81 **The method which the author prefers is to prolapse the rectum and to evert it completely.** Three Babcock's forceps are placed around the edge of the dividend rectum.

82 **The dissection is commenced from the site of division of the rectum working toward the anus.**

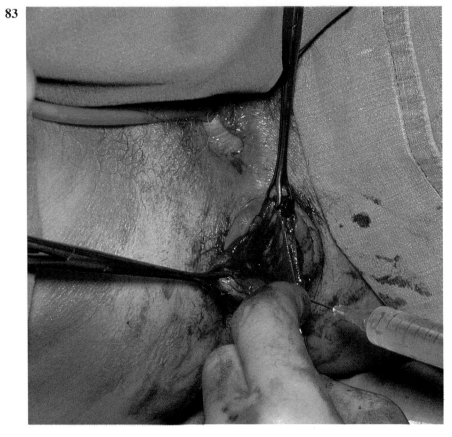

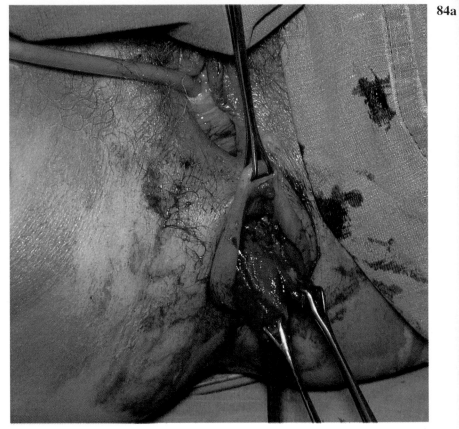

83 A dilute solution of adrenaline is infiltrated into the submucosa to facilitate separation of the layers.

84a and 84b A sheet of diseased mucosa can be dissected off the rectal wall, further infiltrating the submucosal tissues as the dissection progresses.

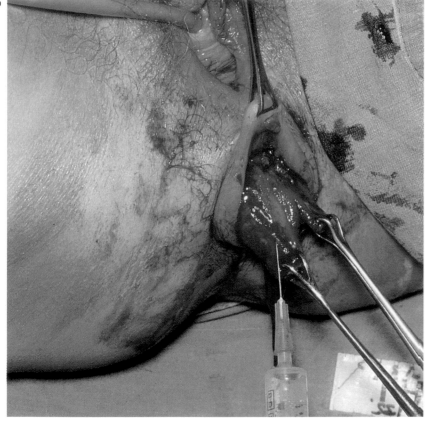

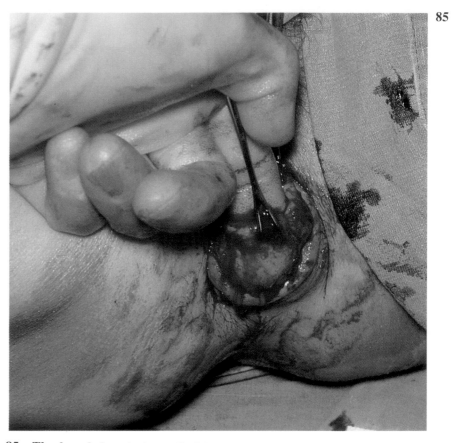

85   The denuded posterior wall of the lower rectum.

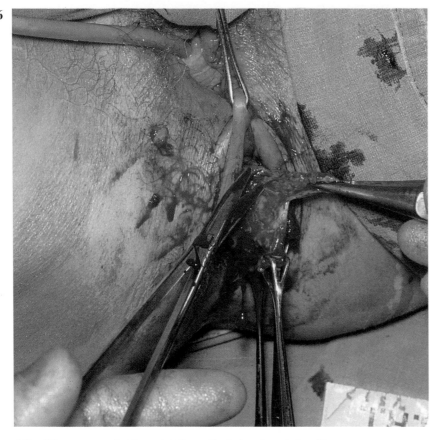

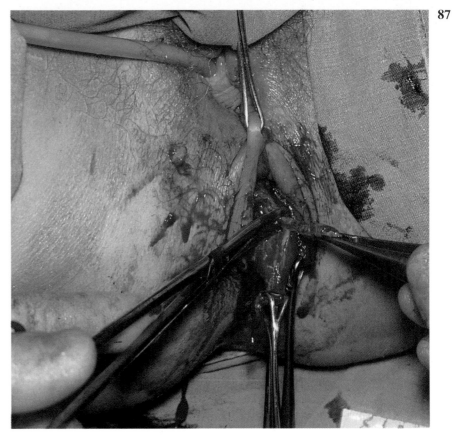

86 The mucosa is dissected from the lateral rectal walls.

87 Stepwise dissection in this way enables the surgeon to complete the mucosal proctectomy.

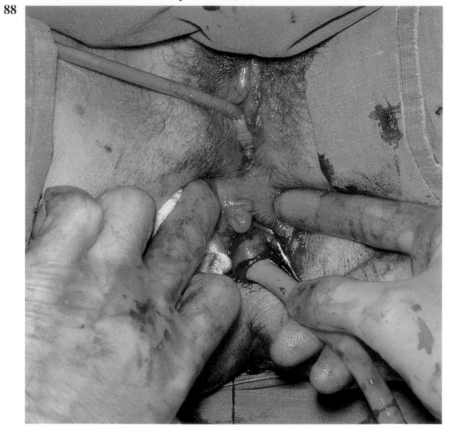

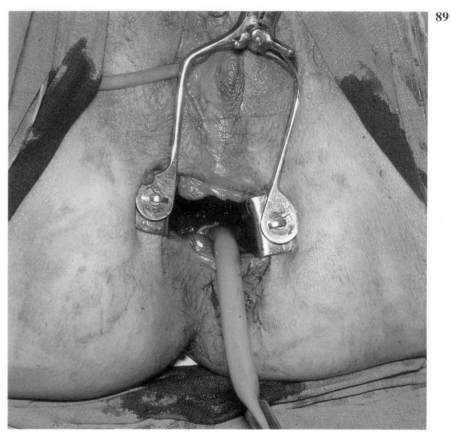

88   The denuded rectum is replaced in the pelvis. The de Pezzer catheter is placed through the rectal remnant and into the perineum.

89   The pouch can be brought down to the level of the anorectal junction in this way.

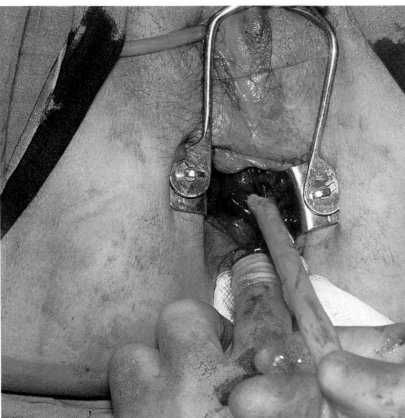

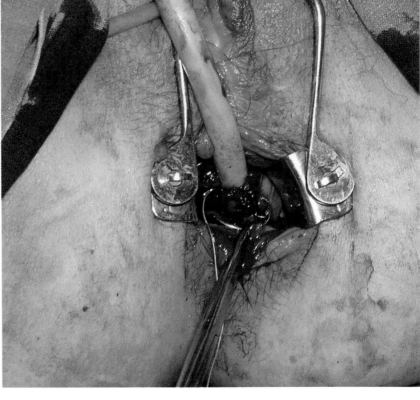

90 The mucosal edges of pouch and the anorectal junction should be apposed without tension prior to suturing.

Caution: Undue tension on the pouch is to be avoided at all costs.

91 and 92 Full-thickness absorbable sutures are placed through the apex of the pouch. A deep bite is inserted into the anorectal junction so as to achieve mucosa to mucosal approximation.

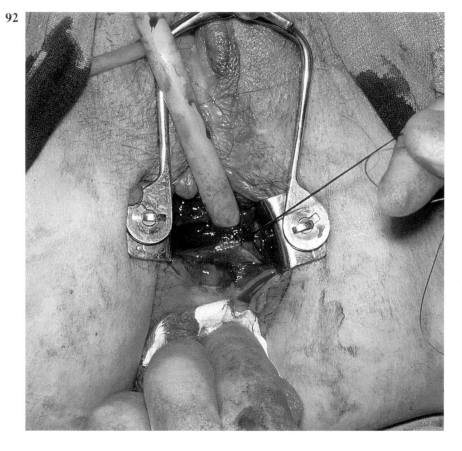

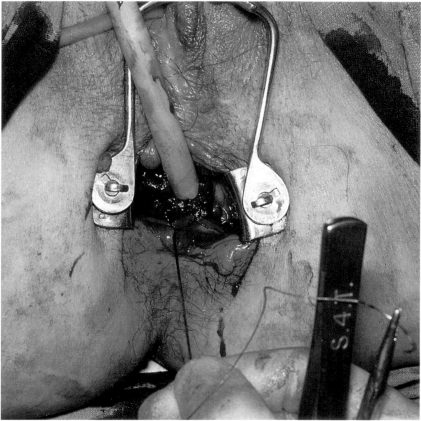

93 The anastomosis progresses around the circumference of the anorectal junction using interrupted sutures.

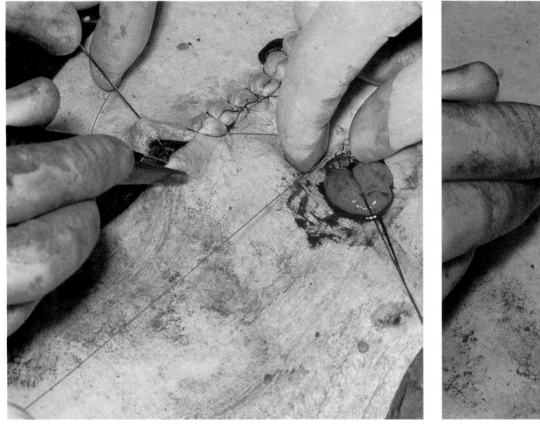

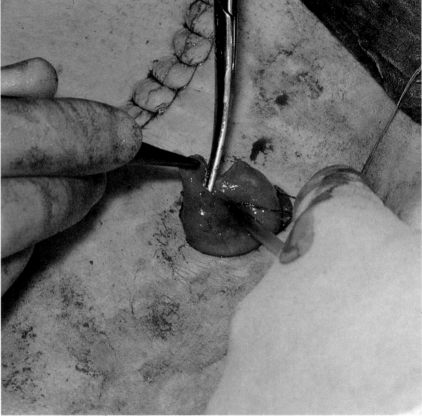

106   Suturing of the skin.

107   Formation of the loop ileostomy.

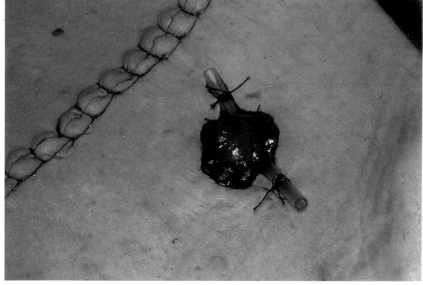

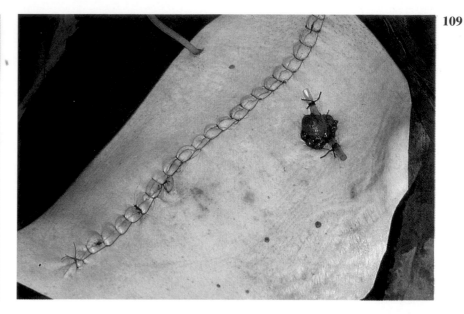

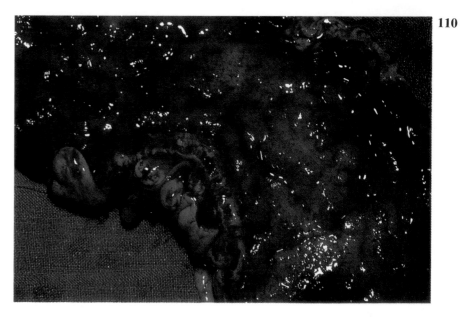

108   The loop ileostomy is sutured over a bridge of plastic tubing. The proximal (draining) component of the ileostomy is made as prominent as possible and the efferent limb is sutured flush with the skin. This is done in an attempt, as far as possible, to avoid skin contamination with the ileal effluent.

109   The completed operation.

110   The mucosa of the excised specimen showing severe ulcerative colitis.

Index